MW01129670

How to Pass the CPA Exa
On the First Try

Kary R. Shumway, CPA

Edited by Jeanne L. Shumway (aka mom)

Copyright © 2015 by Kary R. Shumway

So you want to pass the CPA exam? Do you think you can pass each section on the first try? I didn't think I could either, but I did. The techniques and approach outlined in this guide worked for me, and it is my sincere belief that they can work for you, too. With good preparation, you can pass the CPA exam on the first attempt.

I readily admit that the road to the CPA exam will be a long and tedious one, filled with extensive study, time and effort on your part. But this is a unique journey that you will remember your entire life. The payoff for passing the exam will benefit your entire professional career and you will then hold the coveted letters of our profession: CPA. I did it. So can you.

Now, let's get to work.

Although I had taken business courses in college and held a degree in Business with an Accounting concentration, I had never seriously considered becoming a CPA. It had always seemed too difficult to achieve, and I wasn't even sure that I wanted a career in public accounting.

Then, one day in the early spring, I was shopping at a bookstore with my wife and my parents. I saw a reference book on how to prepare for the CPA exam and immediately a light went on in my head – *I need to do this*. I was in my early twenties, working in a small office for a management company while trying to figure out what I was going to do for my career. I bought the reference book, went outside and sat down at a small café table. And as my wife and parents were eating lunch, it was here that I announced, "I'm going to take the CPA exam."

I said it out loud and that made it real. I believed I would *take* the exam, but I wasn't quite sure at that point if I would ever *pass* the test.

The months after my announcement were filled with reading study guides, taking practice tests, and re-taking courses on auditing and accounting (to learn what I had not paid enough attention to in college). There were many times that I doubted myself and my ability to complete the preparation for the exam, let alone pass the test. But I kept working at it, and before I knew it, exam day had arrived.

The exam was held about an hour's drive from our apartment. Since the test started early, I decided to stay in a hotel nearby, rather than get up early and risk being late. I thought this was a prudent move, but it turned out that my nerves and the 'hotel noises' kept me tossing and turning all night. When I did wake up on exam morning, I was tired, foggy headed and sure that I had ruined my chance to perform well on the test. All my practice and hard work had come down to this day, and I had messed it up before I had even sharpened my number 2 pencil.

The parking lot at the exam location was filling up with cars when I arrived and people were standing around in small groups. They were smiling, happily chatting away with one another. I sat in my car, broke into a cold sweat and pulled out my study note cards. I prayed that I could absorb just a few more bits of information, and that these last seconds of studying would mean the difference between pass or fail. Panic was beginning to set it in. After a few more minutes of futile cramming, I headed inside the building and found a large classroom filled with desks. Back in school again, here we go.

The exam started the way you might expect: the proctor reviewed the time that would be allotted for each section, and the various list of do's and don'ts. The test packets were handed out, my number 2 pencil was poised and ready. And then it was time to begin...

The time between exam completion and receipt of the grades was almost three months. The waiting was absolute torture. In spite of all the test prep and pressure I had put on myself, I seriously doubted my chances for success. I wanted to continue studying during this three month interlude, so that I could re-take those portions of the exam that I didn't pass as soon as possible. But I didn't know yet which sections to study – for all I knew, I had flunked all four parts and would have to study everything, all over again. The waiting was brutal.

Then one day I came home from work to find a letter from the

Board of Accountancy. It was in one of those perforated envelopes, the ones that you have to gently tear off the top, and then ease out the thin paper which, in this case, held the answer to the question: how badly did I screw up this test?

I went upstairs and closed the door to our bedroom. This letter opening had to be done alone, in private, so I could deal with any messy emotions should that be necessary, without subjecting my wife to the gruesome scene. I opened the letter and gently eased out the thin paper that held the grades. My plan was to squint my eyes and slowly reveal one grade at a time. I looked at the first grade, Auditing, and saw with relief that I had passed that section. I looked at the second grade, Financial Accounting, the hardest section which I had no prayer of passing. Amazingly, I had passed that section as well. By this point, since I had already exceeded my expectations by passing the two most difficult sections, I pulled out the entire paper revealing all the grades. I had passed every section of the CPA exam on the first try. This was unbelievable, how did I pull this off? Stay tuned, because that's what this guide is all about.

I believe the information in these pages will help you pass the CPA exam. I encourage you to use these ideas and determine what works best for you. If you like an idea, use it. If you don't like it, toss it out and move on to the next idea. This is not a magic formula or a recipe that needs to be followed word for word, but rather a set of ideas and strategies that you can use to achieve your goal. It worked for me, and I sincerely hope it will work for you as well.

You've Got to Want it

Why do you want to be a CPA? You need to know why, and want it badly enough to put in the time and effort to prepare for and pass the exam.

When I decided to take the exam, it was a flash of inspiration, and not a conscious choice. I suppose the idea had been growing in my head until that one day when it just blossomed and I knew it was time. When that time finally did come, I knew why I wanted it – I wanted a career, I wanted the credentials, I wanted the knowledge and I wanted the recognition. I knew the letters would open doors for me, and they did. A college degree is important, but it doesn't seem to guarantee much other than meeting the first requirement on a job posting. But having the letters CPA after your name? That's a fast pass to some of the better finance jobs on the market. The letters represent proficiency, they represent success, they represent having demonstrated that you can complete and pass one of the more rigorous professional exams out there. The CPA designation is a badge of honor, and it's a badge that I wanted badly to wear.

There is a certain prestige associated with being a CPA. Many times in my career people have said, "Oh, you're a CPA". In other words, you're not just some guy who calls himself an accountant or a Controller or a CFO, you're actually a CPA. The letters mean something to others, and it will mean a great deal to you. I always get a sense of pride and accomplishment when I hear people comment on the fact that I'm a CPA. I think back to the sacrifices and hard work that led to passing the exam and realize it was all worth it.

I wanted to pass the exam because I knew how few people

were able to accomplish this. Success rates in recent years have gone up, but when I sat for the exam the pass rate was very low. And then there was the job market reality that this was a tough club to get into and there would be better job pickings for those who passed. The world needed CPA's and demand was outstripping the supply. I may not have learned a great deal in college, but I did understand that if you are good at doing a job that other people need you to do, and that they don't want to do themselves, they will pay you for it. And sometimes, they will pay you a lot.

The American Institute of Certified Public Accountants (AICPA) set it up so that only Certified Public Accountants could provide certain services to businesses, such as Audits or Reviews. A monopoly on who can Audit financial statements: now that's brilliant. Every publicly held company needs an audit every year, and most any other business that seeks a loan from a bank will need financial statements that have been signed off on by a CPA. The work was there, and it would pay well. Most people didn't want to 'do accounting' to begin with, and those that did had to pass a rigorous exam. The supply was limited, the demand was high, and I wanted to strap on my accounting mojo and get in the game.

I wanted to pass the CPA exam because I felt that I had something to prove. My boss at the time was smart, successful, and a little full of himself. "Do you want to make low 20's your whole life?" he would ask me, referring to how little I was paid. I suppose this was his was his way of giving me a pep talk, or motivating me somehow. Mostly it just made me want to succeed so I could prove him wrong, and shove it in his face when I passed the exam. The desire to' shove it in someone's face' can be a powerful motivator. I'm not terribly proud of this technique, but it worked for me and kept me going. When I hit a wall when trying to learn a new concept I'd think about him and how sweet it was going to be when I announced that I had passed the exam.

Bottom line: You've got to want it. Make a list of the reasons why you want it. Use these as motivation and inspiration to fuel your fire and desire to continue the work necessary to prepare for the exam. It can be a long road, with many opportunities to simply give up and turn back. You've got to want it, and you've got to want it bad. Most people just don't want it bad enough. Do you?

Commitment

Commit to yourself, and commit to the process. It's a long journey and you will have doubts along the way. When I first decided I would take the exam, I didn't have many doubts, simply because I didn't give it a lot of thought and didn't really know what I was getting myself into. The doubts would come later.

Throughout the hard work and practice, I wondered just about every day whether I would be able to pass the exam. I wasn't smart enough, I wasn't working hard enough, there were so many people who were better at this than I was, what made me think I could do this? It was the **commitment to myself and to my family that kept me going.**

I made a commitment to myself, but also out loud to my wife and parents. I made a promise to them that I would sit for the exam and give it my best effort. That promise sustained me in times of doubt during the studying process - and there were a lot of doubts.

Making a commitment to *someone else* makes a big difference. It's relatively easy to promise yourself you will do something, and then decide it's too hard or too much work and you give up. But when you promise someone else, there's an extra incentive to fulfill the commitment. Maybe that extra incentive is guilt or a sense of responsibility or something else, but regardless it provides a little extra fuel for your fire, especially when your commitment starts to weaken.

One of the beautiful things about life is that each day you get a chance to start over. So **each day, renew your commitment to the goal of passing the CPA exam.** Suppose you had a bad day yesterday, you didn't study, you didn't practice, you ate half a cheesecake and watched five hours of bad TV. That happens. It's not a pretty visual but it does happen. So you move on and you start again the next day. You dust off the crumbs from the cheesecake, you open your notebook, study guide and you dive back in. Momentum is gained and lost countless times throughout any project, and this one will be no different. Commit to starting each day new, regardless of how poorly or unproductive the previous day may have been.

A mentor of mine used to say that being in debt was a good thing, "there's nothing like knowing that you have to pay the mortgage to get you out of bed in the morning". I suggest that you find your own 'mortgage' to motivate you to get out of bed and get studying for the exam. **Find your own reason to commit**, and then get out there and fulfill that commitment.

Overview of the Exam

OK, so you've figured out why you want to sit for the exam and you're prepared to commit to the process. The next step is to look at the structure of the test, so you will understand how best to prepare.

The CPA Exam is a computer-based test made up of four sections, and takes a total of 14 hours for all four parts. You may take each part in any order you choose, as long as you pass all four parts within 18 months. Each of the four sections of the exam is graded on a scale of 0 to 99, and the minimum passing score is 75.

The CPA exam is currently made up of four sections:
- Auditing and Attestation (AUD),
- Business Environment and Concepts (BEC),
- Financial Accounting and Reporting (FAR), and
- Regulation (REG)

Auditing and Attestation (AUD) is 4 Hours in length, covering 90 questions and seven task-based simulations. This section covers the entire auditing process, as well as compilations, reviews and attestation engagements, and the AICPA Code of Professional Conduct.

Business Environment and Concepts (BEC) is 3 Hours, with 72 questions and three written communications tasks. This section covers operations and strategic management, economics, financial management and information technology.

Financial Accounting and Reporting (FAR) is 4 Hours, with 90 questions and seven task-based simulations. This section covers differences between financial statements prepared on a U.S. GAAP basis versus those prepared on International Financial Reporting Standards (IFRS) basis. Governmental and not-for-profit accounting is covered as well.

Regulation (REG) is 3 Hours, with 72 questions and six task-based simulations. This section covers federal taxation and business law, including ethics and professional responsibilities.

In total, the sections make up 14 hours of testing, covering 324 questions, and 23 written or 'task based' simulations.

Being able to sit for just one section of the exam at a time is a big advantage in the studying process. When I sat for the exam it was a two day, 14 hour testing marathon. The entire exam, all four sections, were taken consecutively – two sections on the first day, and two on the second day. At that time, you needed to pass two sections with at least a 75 and get at least a 50 on the other two sections, or you lost out on the whole deal and had to start all over again from zero.

Today, you can focus on one section at a time and you have 18 months over which to pass all four sections. This allows you to spread out your study time and nail down each section in turn before moving onto the next.

Understanding the layout and organization of the exam will give you the information you need to formulate a strategy and plan of attack that works best for you. Most standard review courses will help greatly with your game plan, but it helps to get the 'lay of the land' and a sense as to how the exam itself is organized and presented. This approach will help you focus your study on the specific section of the exam you want to take and pass first.

However you structure your approach, the exam study material covers a huge amount of information. There are so many topics on a wide range of subject areas that it is difficult to know where to begin, let alone how to fully prepare to take the exam.

A useful first step is to use basic problem solving techniques: Break the problem into small pieces, divide and conquer, and then formulate a plan of attack.

But, I'm Not a Good Test Taker...

How do you feel about your abilities when it comes to taking tests? Many people say that they "hate tests" and are thrilled to be done with school and the exams that come with it. If you feel uncertain about your abilities, or you've had some rough experiences with "exam freeze" in the past, there is information here that can help.

As I've mentioned, I am not an accounting or financial genius. I enjoy working with numbers and the challenge of learning. However, I knew that all the studying wouldn't count for much if I was going to freeze up and forget everything as soon as the CPA exam was handed out. I needed a strategy to deal with this possibility.

What causes us to forget information at the very moment we need it most? It is the dreaded Test Anxiety and it creeps in at exactly the wrong time. You study, and cram, and force information into your head. Eventually, you feel that you've got it, you understand and you're ready to go. Then you get into an exam situation and poof, it's not there: you just don't remember the answers, the concepts become jumbled, and you doubt yourself.

What is the source of test anxiety and what can you do about it? Test anxiety may be caused by past negative test taking experiences, poor study habits, fear of the unknown, or some combination of all three. Understanding the root cause of your test anxiety is a good first step towards reducing or eliminating this problem during exam time.

Did you have a bad experience with a test in high school that you still carry with you today? You failed the test back then, you froze up and couldn't remember the information, and your past experience taught you that you may freeze up again. Regaining your test taking confidence is essential prior to sitting for the CPA exam.

Think about how many good test taking experiences you've had. Give yourself some credit, there have to be a lot more positive experiences then negative, otherwise you wouldn't have made it out of high school. Draw upon your positive experiences instead of the disasters. Remember, even visualize, how you felt during those experiences - you were in the flow, you knew the information, you were confident. And that is the key, to restore your confidence in your ability to succeed.

Challenge your limiting beliefs. Limiting beliefs are those thoughts or feelings that keep you from achieving what you really want. "I'm not a good test taker", "I always freeze up during tough exams", "'I'm just not smart enough to pass this test." These are all limiting beliefs. You've convinced yourself that you can't do it and, as a result, you may turn out to be correct. Would you rather expect the worst, so you won't be disappointed if you fail? Pessimism doesn't get it done. Expect Success. Why not?

Poor study habits contribute to the problem of Test Anxiety as well. What are your study habits? Are you organized? Are you learning and understanding, or simply memorizing? Organize your study area and workspace. Where possible, the area should be quiet, comfortable and free of distractions. Organize your study guides and practice plans. Be ready to study when you sit down to work, rather than spending the first 20 minutes locating and gathering your materials.

Studying for the exam can be a trap of simply 'memorizing' information. Be careful here, because Memorization + Anxiety = Exam Freeze. Some memorization is unavoidable since you have to learn many concepts in the abstract, rather than getting an opportunity for a practical application or use of the material. Where possible, try to learn and understand the concepts, rather than simply forcing yourself to remember them. When you can, anchor the abstract concepts to practical knowledge that you already have.

Fear of the unknown, or not knowing what to expect on the exam also leads to Test Anxiety. With the CPA exam, you know what to expect regarding the structure and number of questions, it's laid out in the previous chapter and is dealt with in detail in any study guide or CPA exam preparation course. The challenge is that you don't know precisely which topics will be covered on the exam and which will be left out. My fear when preparing for the exam was that the material covered would be exactly the material I did not study completely.

The reality is that the scope of the material that could be covered on the exam is so broad, you can't possibly prepare for everything as much as you might like. However, once you understand the topics, structure of the exam, and types of questions asked, you will have a solid footing to combat any fear of the unknown. You know it's a lot of ground to cover, but the turf will be familiar enough to you, so the surprises will be minimal.

Cast out the Anxiety. I have a technique that I use when I feel the fear, anxiety or self-doubt creeping in. I repeat this statement in my head, or out loud if I'm alone: I cast out and further reject fear, anxiety and self-doubt. I cast them out. In their place I cultivate confidence, determination and self-assuredness. As I am thinking this or saying it out loud I literally wave my hand as if to fling the anxiety away – be gone! The key for me is that I have to nip the anxiety in the bud, recognize that it is trying to get hold of me, and then take the upper hand and cast it aside. It is also important to replace the negative anxiety with something positive – self-confidence, determination and assuredness. The anxiety tells me that I can't, the confidence and determination tells me that I can, and I will. Try this if you like. I practice this regularly, and it has done a world of good for me.

Focused Breathing is another technique used to ease the anxiety. There are many books on this topic, but one technique I've found helpful goes like this: get into a relaxed state, close your eyes, breathe slowly and deeply in, then out. Place the tip of your tongue gently on the roof of your mouth, just behind your front teeth. With your mouth open slightly breathe in gently to a count of four, focus on the air filling up your lungs. Hold the breath gently to a count of seven. Keep your mind focused on the air in your lungs, don't allow your mind to wander off on other subjects or concerns, stay right with your breath. Gently let the air out of your lungs to a count of eight, again focusing on the breath passing out of your lungs, through your mouth. Repeat this breathing technique four times consecutively, and then return to breathing normally.

I find that this breathing technique alleviates the anxiety I may be feeling. Often, I find the cause of the anxiety is that I wasn't breathing well at all. The concentrated deep, long and held breaths make me realize that my stomach had been clenched and I was not breathing fully, just taking minimal short, shallow breaths. The brain works on oxygen, and if you don't breathe properly you are not giving your brain what it needs to work at its best. Without the brain getting its optimal levels of oxygen fuel, it is not going to help you much as you attempt to power your way through the CPA exam.

As good as these techniques are, they need to be practiced regularly in order to work properly. It's hard to just whip out a breathing technique you've only tried once and expect that it will solve your anxiety as the test is being handed out. Try these techniques, practice them, and give them a chance to work for you.

Few people actually like to take tests, but that doesn't mean they're not good at it. I know a business person who has passed dozens of certification exams up to the Microsoft master instructor level, and yet she says, "I'm not a good test taker". Clearly, she is a great test-taker, but she just doesn't like taking the tests themselves.

There can be a lot of pressure when taking any test. You may feel that the grade is going to tell you whether you are competent, smart, or worthwhile. You may feel that getting a poor grade determines that you are a failure. Don't make it harder on yourself. There is an old saying that suffering comes from attachment. If you learn to let go of the attachment to an outcome (passing the exam) then the outcome will be better. The outcome will be better because you are focusing on doing your best work in that moment, and not concerned with pass or fail. You are concerned only with preparing, and learning to the best of your ability. I try to remember this every day. It helps tremendously when starting any new, large project and the problem looks so big, and the road to completion so long. How do I start, and how will I ever finish? Then I remember: Let go of the attachment to the outcome, focus on doing my best work, in this moment.

You are good at taking tests, and you will excel when taking the CPA exam. Build your confidence. Believe in yourself. Prepare. Focus on doing your best work, and the outcome will take care of itself.

Routine of Success

Most people have a routine in their day – they wake up, shower, dress, head to school or to work. There is usually an order and predictability to each day. Changing the routine can be difficult, as you are accustomed to the regimen, it's comfortable, and it works for you. However, to be successful in your quest **to pass the CPA exam, you will need to create a routine of doing things that will lead to your success: a *Routine of Success*.**

It seems so obvious, but most people don't adapt this simple plan: in order to succeed you will need to do things that will lead to your success. The challenge is two-fold: first, identify those actions that you need to take in order to create success, and second change your current daily routine to incorporate these success actions.

Examine your current routine and your habits. What do you do that is good for you, and moving you towards your goal of passing the CPA exam? What parts of your routine are counter-productive? An examination of your current routine will help you change up your daily activities and create a routine of success.

Give your routine serious thought, understand the objectives you are trying to achieve and gear your routine to accomplishing the goal. Write down your routine, post it where you can see it. Give it a chance to work and if it after a few weeks it isn't effective then make changes. There are many books and articles on the routines of successful people. **Do some research, and find what works best for you.**

When is the best time of day to study and prepare? Many

advocate that morning is the best time for thinking and absorbing new thoughts, information and ideas. Others believe that late at night, when the day is done and the issues of the day melt away is best for performing at your highest level. I suspect that there is no perfect time, but there must be a regular and consistent time for you to do your preparation.

There is a remarkable amount of material to cover when preparing for the CPA exam. Map out your plan for covering the material. Determine how much time you can commit each day, and each week to properly study the material and give it the focus that it will need. The amount of study time you need to prepare may just be a numbers game that you can work out for yourself. If you determine that you have two months to prepare for a section of the exam, and you feel you need 60 hours of total study time, you can simply do the math and determine how much time you'll need to study each day. Make this the first part of your routine of success, incorporating a set amount of study time into your day. Commit this time each day, and groove it into your new routine.

Your productivity and study effectiveness may fluctuate from one day to the next. Some days the material makes sense, it's easy, and you're making real progress. Other days the information just doesn't stick, it's confusing, you read the same page three times and the frustration sets in. Do the math on how much time you think you'll need in total, but adjust as you go. After several days or a week, you may want to re-assess and determine if that 60 hour estimate is going to get it done.

If you are taking a **CPA review course**, I recommend that you take the course **in a classroom rather than self-study.** This will force a change into your routine, and ensure that you are focused solely on exam preparation during the class, and not studying at home, wondering what is on TV, or whether there is ice cream in the freezer.

A routine of success should include creating strength and wellness in your body and mind. The simple guidance of proper diet, exercise and adequate sleep is so simple, but it works. You've got to breathe properly to feed your brain the oxygen it needs, you've got to eat and sleep properly to support your body. If you want the mind and body clicking on all cylinders during exam day, you need to treat them right.

Once you've identified and eliminated those counter-productive habits from your current routine, and added those productive habits in, you will need to *ritualize* **the new pattern you have created.** Ritualizing the new habits is simply a matter of doing them consistently and repeatedly each day until they are part of your routine.

Write it down, repeat it aloud, and plan ahead to allow for the routine to work. For example, if your plan is to study through your lunch hour, make sure you pack a lunch and aren't spending the first 20 minutes of the lunch hour driving to and from the market to buy a sandwich. Creating the routine of success is a great tool to help you achieve the goal of passing the CPA exam on the first try.

You Need a Professional Review Course

In my opinion taking a review course is **essential to achieve success on the CPA exam.** Initially, I was resistant to the idea, and thought I knew enough of the basics and could get what I needed from study guides and accounting classes. The cost of the review course was high, my bank account was low, and I figured that I could do as good a job of studying and preparing on my own without the aid and expense of yet another class.

I figured wrong. It is crucial that you take a professional review course. Spend the money, invest the time, and commit to the process. These guys know the format of the exam, they gear the study materials to the areas that will most likely be tested, and give you the structure and discipline you will need to navigate the seemingly infinite material that must be crammed into your brain. They separate the wheat from the chaff, as the saying goes, and they allow you to concentrate your time and effort on the truly important elements of exam preparation.

The two big names in review courses are Lambers and Beckers. I took the Lambers course as it was less expensive and offered a more convenient time and location for the classes. I learned more in the three month Lambers course than I did in four years of accounting classes in college. Granted, I was much more focused and goal-oriented than I was in college. Taking the review course several years removed from college was the best thing for me. My priorities had changed, I had my fun and now it was time to buckle down and actually learn something.

The Lambers classes were **primarily focused on 'teaching to the test'** however the approach was rooted in teaching accounting fundamentals first. This method provided a solid foundation to build on and a great refresher on many concepts that I did not learn thoroughly the first time through in college courses. In short, the CPA exam prep course is not a 'quick fix' or gimmick to help you pass the CPA exam, it is a solid education on the subjects you will need to learn for the test, and the process provides knowledge you will retain throughout your career.

Online courses or self-study computer modules are available to help you study at home or anywhere outside the classroom, and they are a great option if you are disciplined enough to follow these on your own. Most people don't have that kind of discipline, which is why **I recommend that you take one of the classroom options rather than online or self-study.** As noted in the Routine of Success, this will force you to make the needed change in your routine, and have a time set aside on a consistent basis to focus on CPA exam preparation.

Another benefit of live classroom training is the **interaction with the instructor** and other students taking the course. Let's face it, most of the material you will be studying in preparation for the CPA exam is not easy to understand. Live classroom instruction gives you the opportunity to ask a question, have a discussion, and get clarity on the answer. In short, it promotes real learning and understanding, which is what you need to pass the CPA exam.

Re-Take Accounting Courses

It is amazing how much you forget. I took the CPA exam several years after I graduated from college and in that time I forgot most of what I had learned in school. That was money well spent! But I had a great time in college and met my beautiful wife, so the investment paid off in other ways.

Anyway, I **strongly recommend that you re-take many of the core accounting and auditing classes** that you didn't pay attention to in college. For me personally, I was much more mature "intellectually" the second time around and I learned a tremendous amount about the subject matter. The first time around, I was not ready to learn the information. I was taking the classes, mostly just trying to survive them and get my degree. When I took the classes again many years later I was invested in learning the material, not for the grade but for the knowledge which I could apply towards the CPA exam and then to a real career in finance or accounting. This investment paid dividends for me and sitting here many years later, I still remember most of what I learned in that second go-round of accounting classes.

Which classes should you take again? Identify the areas where you feel the weakest and consider re-taking those classes. The primary subject matter that I needed to re-learn was auditing. The class itself filled in a lot of gaps and solidified my auditing fundamentals.

Many colleges offer the option to audit a class, rather than enrolling as a student. This can be far less expensive, and in most cases, you don't need the credits. Your goal is knowledge.

Re-taking the course also helped me practice up for the CPA

exam testing experience that was to come. Sitting in classes and taking tests allowed me to shake off the rust that had accumulated since I left college. Since I wasn't taking the course for the purpose of achieving a high grade, the pressure was off and I could focus simply on learning the material. This process really helped me gain confidence in my test-taking abilities, and gave me many opportunities to practice that skill.

Back to Basics

Sometimes, simple just works. I listen to audiobooks on my commute into work, and the Sue Grafton crime mysteries are a favorite of mine. The lead character in the books used an old fashioned approach to crime-solving – she writes down clues and **information on note cards,** using this technique to organize her thoughts and eventually to solve the crime. It works to solve murder mysteries, and it will work to help you pass the CPA exam on the first try.

My technique was to take the key learning areas from each section of the study guides, and summarize the information on note cards. If there was an area that I was having particular trouble with, I found that writing it down on the notecards helped me absorb the information. When forced to summarize the topic, it required that I condense the information to the essential points. This pushed me to uncover what was truly important in the subject matter, and leave out repetitive or un-necessary information.

Initially, it was very difficult to summarize the information and I found myself simply re-writing the entire section of the study guide on dozens of notecards. In time though, the process became easier and soon I was able to distill pages of information down to two or three easy to read notecards.

By writing the summarized information on notecards it made the studying process more portable. It was easy to grab three or four note cards, and drill on the subject matter over and over during lunch or when I had a free moment during the day. This was a helpful tool to use for those topics that just didn't make sense to me the first few times I studied them. The notecards allowed me to repeat the information over and again, focusing only on those topics which needed extra time.

Breaking the problem into smaller parts allowed for the material to be much more manageable and digestible. I wasn't overwhelmed when studying eight or ten note cards, and this made the material much more approachable. An accounting textbook with 400 pages was daunting, but a handful of notecards with a few key sentences on each was much more welcoming. A journey of one thousand steps began with a single note card.

Using the notecards, I could also have my wife quiz me on certain topics. Much like a flash card, I would write the question on one side, and the answer on the other. She would read the question, wrinkle her nose, and comment on how boring this stuff was. I would then take the note cards back and give myself the quiz instead.

The process of writing out the information required that I handle the material repetitively and repeatedly, giving me numerous passes over the same information. Everyone learns differently, and at their own pace, but **repetition is a foundation to all learning.**

Sitting for the Exam - Literally

It is not a coincidence that taking the CPA exam is referred to as "sitting for the exam" because you are literally sitting for three to four hours at a time on each section. When I took the exam, the requirement was to sit for all four sections over a two day period. This was 14 hours of sitting, and test taking over two days. Therefore, **some useful guidance is to *practice* sitting for long periods** of time. You won't need to sit for six or seven hours at a stretch, but you will be planted in that chair for what will feel like an eternity if you don't *practice sitting*.

It's like running a marathon. I know that sounds ridiculous, but there is a certain stamina required for long periods of sitting. **Physically, this can be much more difficult than it would appear**. The mental marathon of a four hour exam is obvious, and clearly much of the guidance here and advice you will receive from study manuals and others who have taken the exam is to get your mind ready, but don't forget the physical toll this will take on you.

Think back to the last time you had to sit on an airplane for three or four hours. Cramped, crowded, not comfortable. It was hot, stuffy and there was no fresh air coming your way for a long time. Now imagine that experience, but this time you have the Financial Accounting and Reporting section of the exam in front of you. You're staring at a four hour exam with the 90 questions and seven task-based simulations. Worse yet, you don't even get the little bag of peanuts or complimentary drink from the beverage cart.

You do get more leg room to work with in the CPA exam room as compared with the plane, but not much. The point here is that you need to practice working and testing yourself in an uncomfortable environment for the full stretch of time. Ease into it. Plant yourself in the chair and do one or two hours straight without getting up. Work your way up to the full four hours. Find out how your body responds.

You will likely start to tighten up after an hour, and start to feel edgy after two hours. Learning some simple stretches and practicing the breathing techniques learned earlier will help you stay sharp. There are numerous stretches you can try, below are a few examples that I've found helpful.

Head turn and neck stretches. Face straight ahead and turn your head to one side without moving your shoulders. Hold the position for ten seconds and feel the tension release from your neck. Do the same, turning your head to the other side. Don't forget to breathe! Next, tilt your head towards your shoulder, without lifting your shoulder. Hold the position for ten seconds. Repeat by tilting your head towards the other shoulder. Go slowly, and feel the tension leaving your neck and shoulders. This is the area that usually tenses up the most when you're hunched over the desk.

Chest stretch. This one really gets the blood flowing. Put your hands behind your head, and squeeze your shoulder blades together, moving your elbows back as far as possible. Take a nice deep breath and hold this position for several seconds. Repeat this stretch several times and breathe in deeply each time.

Lightbulb stretch. Lace your fingers together and stretch high above your head. Inhale as you stretch upward. Your arms and body will resemble a lightbulb, therefore the name of the stretch!

Experiment with different stretches and find out what works best for you. Movement is what is most important to relieve some tension and get the blood flowing so that you can keep your focus and stay energized for the four hour sitting marathon.

Test Yourself Again and Again

Reading and studying the CPA exam material without testing yourself is obviously pointless. Much of the material is abstract and difficult to grasp by simply reading about it. Quizzing yourself regularly and frequently will help reinforce the knowledge you are studying.

Most of your studying will be followed by taking short practice tests – 10 or 20 questions at a time. This is a good way to reinforce the specific subject matter you just learned, but it is not enough. I **highly recommend taking a full section of the CPA exam several times**. This will help you with both the mental and physical approach to the exam and give you a sense as where you need additional work. What was your overall grade? How did you hold up mentally? What strategies will you need to employ if you start to experience exam freeze?

Most professional athletes understand that to excel in their sport they need to 'slow down the game'. In other words they don't panic or become overwhelmed by the pressure. These athletes trust themselves, their training, and their natural ability. This is a solid strategy that can be used when taking the exam, and it's one that worked for me. The CPA exam is a timed test, and this time limit may contribute to the pressure you feel to hurry through the questions so you don't run out of time. However, this is where it becomes important when you practice taking tests that you time yourself.

Time yourself and make the conditions similar to what you will experience in the actual exam setting. John Wooden, the famous UCLA basketball coach used to say 'be quick, but don't hurry'. That is a succinct and appropriate way to describe how you should approach the questions on the exam. **Be methodical in your approach.**

Each section of the CPA exam has a time limit, so when you test yourself make sure that you set a timer and **stick to the time limit.** This will allow you to practice pacing yourself, and determine the proper rhythm you will need in the actual exam. You'll get a feel for when you are falling behind the pace, and need to push yourself a bit faster. Or you'll realize you are speeding ahead and can slow down and give extra time and attention to the questions. **Timing yourself will help develop your pace and rhythm**, so that you use the full allotted time to your best advantage. No points for finishing early!

As discussed previously, the CPA exam involves long periods of sitting, without the option to go outside after a few hours and get some fresh air. Simulate the actual conditions of the exam. Push yourself to sit for the full portion of the test. Practice your 'seated stretches' to keep the blood circulating properly, and work on your breathing to keep the oxygen flowing to your brain where you need it most.

Calculate your overall grade. With all the topics and concepts flying around it is easy to lose sight of the fact that you do in fact need a passing score to pass the CPA exam! **Calculate your grade, but don't over-react to the result.** You will test yourself again and again, this is just the first go round. The grade is a good indicator of how ready you may be to sit for that section of the CPA exam, or whether you need to go back and drill on specific topics. Examine where you did well and where you did poorly. Adjust or fine tune your Routine of Success as necessary to make the needed improvements.

Put a little pressure on yourself during your practice test to simulate the pressure you will feel when it is time for the real exam. This pressure will help you determine if 'exam freeze' is going to be an issue for you. If you do experience this during your practice test, re-read the earlier chapter on how to combat the exam freeze. This is a good opportunity to practice the techniques discussed earlier.

Hone your test taking skills. You are in this for the knowledge and for the CPA credentials, but at the end of the day you need a passing score on the exam to get your letters. Testing in small sections of 10 or 20 questions is a great way to reinforce specific topics or concepts. **Putting it all together and simulating a four hour exam is very important** to hone your test taking skills for the real exam, and ensure that on exam day you will be confident, prepared, and ready to do your best work.

The Art of War

Sun Tzu was an ancient military strategist who wrote The Art of War, the classic work on military strategy and tactics. While you are not going to war, you will be in a battle of wits with the CPA exam and many of the strategies from this classic book can be applied in your preparation for the exam.

The Art of War consists of thirteen chapters covering topics such as Laying Plans, Tactical Dispositions and the Use of Spies. Below is a summary of each chapter, and how it may be applied and used in your *battle plan* for passing the exam.

Laying plans. Research and planning are the key to any endeavor. This involves conducting a detailed assessment and planning of your mission, calculating your chances of victory, and tracking and monitoring your progress.

Waging War. Success requires winning decisive engagements quickly. Sun Tzu said "Let your main object be victory, not lengthy drawn-out campaigns." Your goal is to pass the exam not become a career student. Focus your energy on the task at hand. Do not allow yourself to become distracted from your goal. Study hard and efficiently.

Attack by stratagem. The source of strength is unity, not size or superior brain power. Your strength will come from your unwavering focus on the single unified goal of passing the CPA exam. You may not be the brightest bulb, but if you concentrate your entire focus, shine your light on your one goal, you will succeed. "If you know neither the enemy nor yourself, you will succumb in every battle". Be honest with yourself about your strengths and weaknesses. Be firm in your resolution to understand what will be expected of you on the exam.

Tactical dispositions. Recognize strategic opportunities, such as the CPA exam preparation courses, and use them to your advantage. Strategically plan your studies and your efforts for maximum efficiency and results by focusing on those topics which are most likely to be tested. Do not create opportunities for the 'enemy' by wasting time, being disorganized in your preparations or losing focus.

Energy. Momentum is critical in achieving your goal. Just as the use of creativity and timing in building an army's momentum is vital, so too is creating momentum in your studying, learning and preparation for the CPA exam.

Weak points and strong. Opportunities come from the openings caused by the relative weakness of the enemy in a given area. Understand the elements of the CPA exam, and where there are relative weaknesses. Are there areas or sections that are easier than others for you? Exploit these first.

Maneuvering. Maneuvering with an army is advantageous; with an undisciplined multitude, most dangerous. Discipline and organization in your study habits is critical to success.

Variation in tactics. Flexibility and adaptability are critical in battle. You must learn how to respond to shifting circumstances and overcome them. You may be thrown a curve ball on the exam, a question or series of questions you did not anticipate. Adapt, use your critical thinking, and work through the problem in a logical manner.

The army on the march. You will encounter different

situations in new enemy territories and must learn how to respond. The CPA exam is held in an offsite location, one that is likely not familiar to you. Prepare yourself for potentially adverse conditions.

Terrain. There are three areas of general resistance: distance, dangers and barriers. Distance: it is a long road to complete the exam. Dangers: self-doubt, disorganization, lack of focus. Barriers: time, resources, effort. Examine and be mindful of these areas of resistance.

The nine situations. Here Sun Tzu discussed the different types of battlegrounds – from mountains to marshes and narrow gorges. We are most concerned with 1) knowing how to get to the testing center on the day of the exam and 2) dressing properly for the occasion.

Prior to exam day, visit the location where the exam will be held and become familiar with the surroundings. You don't want any surprises on testing day. Be sure you know exactly how to get to the testing location, and how long it will take to get there. Don't rely on the GPS. How many times has the GPS led you astray and delivered you efficiently and directly to the wrong address? Sun Tzu did not have GPS, but if he did he would not rely on it.

The Elements. Your reconnaissance mission should include a visit to the building and classroom where the test will be held. What kind of temperatures can you expect, what kind of lighting and atmosphere. Minor details you say? Imagine a scenario where it's 90 degrees in August, and you arrive at the testing location in short sleeves and shorts, only to discover the air conditioning in the classroom is set at an icy 64 degrees. That is four hours of exam time chattering your teeth and thinking about how cold you are. It's a distraction you can and should avoid.

Arrive early. *Sun Tzu said: Whoever is first in the field and awaits the coming of the enemy, will be fresh for the fight; whoever is second in the field and has to hasten to battle will arrive exhausted.* On the day of the exam, it is to your advantage to arrive early, await the start of the exam, and you will be fresh for the fight.

The attack by fire. In battle, it is vital to select the proper weapons for the specified target. During the CPA exam, your *weapon* will be the computer, and your ability to navigate the keyboard and the mouse. Unless you have been living under a rock for the last twenty years, you should be well acquainted with a keyboard and mouse, and prepared to deploy these weapons in battle.

The use of spies. The importance of developing good information sources and the management of this information cannot be underestimated. Gather data. Talk to others who have taken the exam. Develop a relationship with your CPA preparation course instructor. Manage and organize your information to your greatest advantage.

These tactics are helpful tools that you can use in preparation for exam day. The goal is to eliminate distractions or unexpected surprises so that you can give your full attention and energy to the exam itself. The more variables that you can eliminate on exam day, the better you will be prepared to achieve your goal of passing the CPA exam.

Remember it for Life

Sitting for and passing the exam is the immediate goal, but the knowledge and understanding that you will acquire during this process will last you a lifetime.

As I was studying, I was consciously trying to avoid memorizing information. I wanted to learn it and make it part of the fiber of my accounting being. I can tell you that after years of being a CPA in public practice, the material that I learned when studying for the exam has benefitted me professionally for my entire career. Remember this when you are drilling facts into your head and wondering if you'll ever need this stuff after the exam is over with. The information you learn while preparing for the exam will fuel your career long after you hang that CPA certificate on the wall.

Lessons Learned

In theory we all grow older and wiser. Growing older just happens, but growing wiser requires a little more work. Since taking the CPA exam, I have learned a few lessons that I would like to share with you.

Believe in yourself. Henry Ford said "whether you think you can or think you cannot, you are right". Believe you can pass the exam. I've found that believing in myself has to be practiced and has to be a regular reminder. It is too easy to be overcome by the perceived setbacks, small failures and mis-steps of daily life. Remind yourself every day that you believe in yourself and your abilities. Focus on your steps forward, your small wins, and the little improvements you have made. You can choose to think you can or you cannot. Make it a little easier on yourself as you are preparing for the CPA exam, think that you can, and believe in yourself.

Ask for help. Preparing for the exam should not be done in isolation. Where possible, find a study group, or at least one other partner that you can work with and ask for help when you need it. If you decide to take an exam preparation course, ask the class instructor for help if you don't understand the subject matter. Most people are willing to share what they know, and want to help you succeed. But most of the time, we just don't ask. Don't suffer in silence, ask for help.

Get a Mentor. After I passed the exam, and began working at a CPA firm I was assigned a 'mentor'. For the next two years, my mentor would work with me on the finer points of audit engagements, tax work and general interpersonal relationships with clients. This mentorship was one of the most rewarding experiences of my professional career. As I look back, I believe that if I had sought out a mentor earlier on in my career, when I was preparing for the CPA exam, my experience would have been so much better, so much deeper in understanding.

How do you find a mentor? Simply look around you. Who do you admire? Who do you have a great respect for and want to learn from? It could be someone you already know personally, or someone you only know by name and reputation. Determine what it is you are looking for. Do you want someone to help you in preparing for the CPA exam specifically, or are you looking for someone to prepare you for your career beyond the exam? Be clear about what you want to learn and have your future mentor teach you. Approach the person. Many opportunities in life are achieved by merely asking for what you want.

Get experience in Public accounting. After I passed the CPA exam, I interviewed at several public accounting firms. Initially, I wanted to work at one of the big CPA firms, and was offered a job at what was then Coopers & Lybrand. Taking the job would have required moving to the city, and this was not a move I was ready to make at that time. I ended up taking a position at a much smaller firm with a professional staff of ten people. Although this firm was small in comparison to Coopers, it was a good sized firm for the area I worked in, and it provided me exposure to a wide variety of engagements in different industries. The experience at that 'small' firm was invaluable and I carry with me today the lessons learned there.

Never try, never win. I have an old picture of my father standing next to a large boulder engraved with the words "Never Try, Never Win." For some reason that image and that quote have stuck with me over the years. My dad would say these words whenever one of the kids would want to try something new, or if we weren't sure if we could do something. "Never Try, Never Win!" he would say with a smile. It was never heavy handed or preaching, it was just a light-hearted, good natured suggestion to give it your best try, and you might just win.

Do you want to take and pass the CPA exam? It starts with the plan, the practice, and the dedication. The reward of putting the letters *CPA* after your name is wonderful. The knowledge you gain along the way will last you a lifetime. I wish you the best of luck in your journey and in your future career as a CPA.

41568024R00027

Made in the USA
Middletown, DE
17 March 2017